BREAST FEEDING
MADE EASY

Breast Feeding Made Easy

How To Breastfeed For Mothers Of Newborns

Debra Harper

The information provided in this book is designed to provide helpful information on the subjects discussed. This book is not meant to be used, nor should it be used, to diagnose or treat any medical condition. For diagnosis or treatment of any medical problem, consult your own physician. The publisher and author are not responsible for any specific health or allergy needs that may require medical supervision and are not liable for any damages or negative consequences from any treatment, action, application or preparation, to any person reading or following the information in this book. References are provided for informational purposes only and do not constitute endorsement of any websites or other sources. Readers should be aware that the websites listed in this book may change.

TABLE OF CONTENT

Start Breast Feeding

As you hold your precious baby for the very first time, you should put his lips to your breast. Even though mature milk has not been developed yet, the breasts are in the production of colostrum - a substance which helps protect your baby from infections. Don't panic if your baby has difficulty in finding or staying on your nipple. It is very normal.

The art of breast feeding (yes, it is an art) requires tremendous amount of patience and practice. You can't expect to be an expert on first attempt and you must seek for advice or have a medical practitioner show you what to do. Once you start doing it, bear in mind that nursing wouldn't be painful. Once your baby latches on your breasts, pay attention to how your breasts feel.

If it hurts, gently break the suction and try again. Try nursing more frequently as the more you nurse, the quicker your mature milk would come in and the more it will produce. Ideally, the target should be 10 to 15 minutes per breasts, of around 10 times a day.

When the baby cries, it is a signal that he is hungry. However, you should always look to feed the baby before he even starts crying. During the first few days of the newborn, it is essential to wake your baby to start the breast feeding. The baby would even end up falling asleep during the feeding. To make sure that your baby is eating regularly, wake him up if it has been more than four hours since his last 'meal'.

When the baby first starts, it may take more than forty minutes or even longer. Therefore, you should look to be comfortable. If you are sitting in a place where you would be bothered, it makes the process very difficult. This guide is about that - to teach you how to be comfortable and the factors that you would consider.

Why You Should Breast Feed

Research has tried to find what makes breast milk perfect for babies' development. There has been years of research being done on this subject as we know that during the baby years is when they need to eat a lot of good nutrients.

Researchers have discovered that there are more than two hundred compounds used in fighting infection, aid digestion and assist the immune system. Regardless of what nature-made ingredients, science simply can't do the same thing.

There are several long term benefits from breast feeding which includes reduced risk of asthma, obesity and some form of child cancer. As the researchers do more studies, it has been found that breast milk is extremely good for the development of the child. It not only makes the baby healthier, but also makes them smarter. Studies have shown that babies who are breast-fed tend to be smarter than babies fed with formulas.

Simply speaking, breast feeding helps with the right nutrients and support brain growth. Every mother should think deeply about this. Besides this, breast feeding doesn't just help the baby but the mother as well. When a mother breast feed, hormones are released which help curb blood loss post-delivery and assist in shrinking the uterus to its normal size.

Over the long term, mothers would also have a lower risk of premenopausal breast cancer. This cancer is something which strikes women under 50 years of age. The benefits of breast feeding can be shown just three to six months and increase even more when breast feeding continues.

Breast feeding is indeed a powerful liquid. It is much better than formula or any scientific creation that would be created. Making a commitment to breast feed your child is the best thing you can do, not only for your child but for you as well.

Besides all these physical benefits, there are other benefits as well. This includes saving costs of buying the formulas. Formulas are getting more and more expensive. When you start breast feeding your child, you would be able to save a tremendous amount of money.

However, no benefit is more important than allowing the baby to bond with the mum. The breast feeding process is a very intimate process. In fact, research has proven that those mothers who breast feed their children tend to be closer than them compared to those people who don't.

It is clear that breastfeeding holds various benefits. In the next chapter, I would explain the wonderful process in which breast milk is made.

How Is Breast Milk Made

Any women who have been pregnant would notice a metamorphosis in their bra cups. There are certain physical changes like tender and swollen breasts, which is the most important indication that you have conceived.

Experts believe that this color change at the areola can be very useful for breast feeding. This is an indication of the changes that are happening biologically. The placenta which is developing would stimulate the release of progesterone and estrogen. This release help stimulate the biological system. This assists the lactation process.

Before a woman gets pregnant, the larger portion of your breasts is made up of a combination of milk glands, supportive tissue and fat. The truth is your swollen breasts had been preparing for pregnancy from the time you are in your mother's womb. Before a woman is even born, milk ducks have already been formed.

However, the mammary glands aren't kick started until a women reaches the age of puberty. The flood of female hormone estrogen would make them grow and swell. During pregnancy, this process moves faster. When the baby arrives, glandular tissue would have replaced majority of the fat cells and that is the reason why they breasts are bigger.

If a woman takes time to measure their breast, they may even realize that each breast is actually 1.5 pounds heavier than previously. Among the breasts is an intricate network of channels known as milk ducts.

Those pregnancy hormones would mean that those ducts would increase in both size and number. The ducts would be branched off into smaller canals around the chest wall known as ductules. Located at the end of each duct is a cluster of smaller sacs known as alveoli.

This cluster of alveoli is known as the lobule. A cluster of lobule is known as a lobe. Every breast has around 15 lobes, with a milk duct for every lobe.

The breast milk is produced inside the alveoli, surrounded by tiny muscles with squeeze the glands and push the milk out into the ductules. This leads to a bigger duct which widens the milk pool directly below the areola.

These milk pools act as reservoirs which hold the milk until your baby start sucking it through the nipples. This is how breast feeding is done - the power of Mother Nature, producing such an amazing 'milk-factory' inside the human body.

The Nursing Area

As you reach the third trimester, it is expected that most pregnant women would start having nursing bras, breast pads and loose button-down shirts to prepare for the next few months. While breast feeding, you could also have your own personal area.

This is to ensure that you are comfortable and it should reflect your personality. This may be in a living room if you like to be around family members or a quiet place in your bedroom if you want solitude during the breast feeding.

It is ideal to have an extra chair to ensure that your family members or friends could keep you needed when needed. However, most people prefer a quiet place because they perceive breast feeding as a very intimate activity. You could simply close the door, dim the lights and breast feed. Preferably, if you can get one, find a reclining sofa to ensure that you are comfortable.

During the breast feeding, you would be sitting on the chair for several hours a day. This would ensure that you are comfortable. Find for one which offers a certain shoulder and back support, together with wide arm rests. To support your underfoot, you could use a footstool or simply a stack of pillows.

When you raise your legs and feet to push your baby to your breast, it would avoid a possible backache. Pillow your neck, feet, arms and back. This would ensure that you are as comfortable as possible.

For additional comfort, find a special made nursing pillow which circles your waist. Try finding a small table or stand beside your chair would also help. This should be within arm's length from your breast feeding chair. The table should be wide enough to hold a coaster and a glass of liquid.

Certain women prefer drinking from a straw while other prefer drinking for a glass. Besides drinks, you may also want to have certain snacks. Make sure it is healthy, like nuts, fresh fruits or crackers to replace the energy you use. Your baby may be a slow eater or a baby with big appetite.

Therefore, having snacks beside you ensure that you won't feel hungry during the lengthy process.

Besides that, you can even read a book or do some crossword puzzles to ensure that you are occupied while your baby is full. Find for anything that would possible interest you to make sure that you aren't bored.

Food To Avoid While Breast Feeding

There is a myth that women could eat anything they want during breast feeding. However, this isn't entirely accurate. Certain strongly-favored foods would change the taste of the breast milk. Babies may enjoy different varieties of breast milk flavors but at times, the baby may be cranky after you eat certain food.

Simply put, the food you eat would affect the taste of the milk from your breasts. If you notice your baby unhappy after drinking, simply avoid the food.

Among the food you should try to avoid include spices, garlic, chili, lime, chocolate and gassy vegetables. You may have a cup of coffee each day, but drinking too much caffeine could interfere with your baby's sleep. Bear in mind that caffeine is found in other beverages like sodas, tea and even in some medication.

When it comes to alcoholic beverages, it is recommended to keep it to a bare minimum. Try not to drink more than a drink as it would increase the alcohol level in your blood and this would put alcohol into your breast milk.

However, don't simply cut out any food from your diet. Talk to your doctor about this first. The reason is that if you simply omit any food, there is a possibility that it would cause a nutritional imbalance in your body and affect your breast milks as well. For a more professional consultancy, see a nutritionist. They may advice to take certain other foods or to take nutritional supplements.

Choosing A Breast Pump

The production of breast milk works on a simple principle of supply and demand. As your baby consumes more milk, your body would need to make more milk. As such, breast pumps are normally used to ensure the continued production of breast milk when you couldn't feed your baby when you are travelling or out of town.

There are various types of breast pumps. It could be battery-operated, hand-operated, semi-automatic or self-cycling electric. Hand pumps are generally recommended because it allows you to use the strength of your arm. This doesn't just allow you to pump milk, but also allows you to get some exercises.

Besides that, there are also pumps which use your leg and foot muscles for breast pumping. This is especially better for those mothers with carpal tunnel syndrome as they would train their arms as well.

Battery operated breast pumps are the best for women who have a consistent supply of milk and desire to pump once or twice a day. The pumps use batteries to create suction and this minimizes and forms of muscle fatigue. However, these types of electric pumps are more expensive even though it is more efficient.

You could rent these battery operated pumps if you need to. Electric pumps can be easily plugged to an outlet and you can use it frequently as and when you like. Hospital grade pumps, meanwhile, are the best in ensuring the milk supply. You can rent or purchase them based upon your needs.

How To Use A Breast Pump

Similarly to breast feeding, using a breast pump is a skill as well. It is very normal for mothers to be able to pump only a few drops of milk when using a breast pump. It is important to have the right knowledge and practice them well. From here, the mother would be more efficient. When using a breast pump, ensure:

- That you read the instructions carefully and thoroughly
- Your breast pumps are sterilized carefully before using it
- If your doctor feels it is important, sterilize the kit every day

- After using it, make sure that you wash the pump in warm soapy water. Rinse with hot water and dry it on a clean towel. You don't have to clean the plastic tube unless you get milk on it. However if there is milk on it, make sure that you dry and drain it thoroughly.
- If you use an electric pump, set the suction level to the lowest. Start low because it isn't something that you could get used to immediately.

Tips For Breast Pumping

- Massage your breast and gently stimulating your nipples as this helps stimulate an easier let down for your baby.

- Make sure to always relax while you are performing the breast massages. Many mothers prefer to close their eyes and imagine their baby is in their arms. If the mother is more relaxed, the easier the letdown would be and the easier the milk would be dispensed.

- First attempts at breast pumping are difficult. Consider them as practice sessions for learning how to use the breast pump.

- Start with short pumps at the start. When using a hand pump, quick and short pumps at the beginning is more stimulating and imitates better the way a baby breast feeds. Once the milk starts to flow freely; longer and steadier strokes are more efficient and not so tiring.

- When first learning to pump, practice for around five minutes on a side at least twice a day. Choose the least stressful part of your day for pumping as it could be a very tiring activity.

- You need to realize that the pump is your friend and it is very important to relax before using it. To relax, the mother can do several things like playing games, talking to some of her friends, read books or simply any other thing up to her. The process of breast feeding can be extremely long when first starting and simply watching the collection bottle wouldn't help. It would probably put more stress on the mother instead.

The First Six Weeks Of Your Baby

Without a doubt, breast milk is the best food to give your baby because of its completeness and nutrition. According to a research, there are a minimum of 400 nutrients in it, including hormones and disease fighting compounds that can't be found in formulas. The most powerful thing about breast milk is that the nutritional compound of it changes as your baby grows older.

Besides building the brain, there are also the benefits of fighting infection. No formula can ever match breast milk. Besides that, the mother can also create a special bond between her and the baby. During this nursing the baby thrives on cuddling, holding and human contact. Without a doubt, the mother would feel the same as well.

The atmosphere during breast feeding is very important. Generally speaking, it would take up to 45 minutes and you should choose a comfortable sport for it. This is extremely important during the early days of the baby when you are still trying to get used to it. Go to somewhere quiet if you are easily distracted by noise. Besides that, you should hold your baby in the right position so that your body wouldn't be sore.

It remains the best thing to support the back of the baby's head with your hand.

When supporting the baby, a nursing pillow is of great help and you should never feed the baby until both of you are comfortable.

When the baby latches onto the breasts, pay attention to how you feel. His mouth should cover most of the areola below your nipple and the nipple should be comfortable in your baby's mouth.

Some mothers find breast feeding difficult to learn. It is normal to feel discouraged at the beginning, but you need to realize that you are not the only one uncomfortable with it. When starting, everyone would feel different. It depends a lot on the mother and the situation she is in.

Like it or not, breast feeding is something which takes practice. Give yourself some time to ensure that it becomes natural for you. Take one feeding at a time and don't stress yourself out if you have a bad day.

Bear in mind that any problems that you face are temporary and if you give it enough time, you could be like a pro within six weeks of postpartum checkup. However, it may be a roller-coaster ride in the first six weeks.

It is impossible to know everything before you begin. That is where the practice would help you become better and the more you breast feed, the more you would learn. Besides that, the bond that you have with your baby is invaluable, something to last you a lifetime.

Using Breast Compression

The main purpose of breast compression is to ensure that the milk flows to the baby once the baby no longer drink on his own. Besides that, compression would also stimulate a letdown reflex and cause a more natural letdown to happen. Breast compression is also very useful when:

- You are feeding a baby who falls asleep very fast
- There is a recurrent of blocked ducts
- Poor weight gain in the baby
- There is colic in the breast-fed baby
- Feedings which are too long

- You have sore nipples

When everything is well, breast compression may not be necessary. If everything is alright, the mother should allow the baby to feed finish on the first side. If the baby wants some more, offer the other breast.

Steps To Using Breast Compression

1. Gently hold your baby with one arm, preferably your stronger arm.
2. Hold your breast with your other arm, thumb on a side of the breast while your finger are on the other, far back from the nipple
3. Look out as the baby is drinking. You don't have to ensure that the baby

catches every suck but the baby would get more milk if he or she drinks with an open pause.

4. As and when the baby nibbles or is no longer drinking, you should compress the breast. It doesn't have to be hard until it hurts. With breast compression, the baby should be drinking again.

5. Maintain the pressure until the baby no longer needs to drink with compression and then gently release the pressure. When the baby doesn't stop sucking with the compression; release, wait for a little while before compressing again.

6. Releasing pressure allows your hand to rest and allow the breast milk to

flow easily to the baby again. If the baby stops sucking when you release the pressure, he would start sucking again once he taste the milk. If the baby starts to suck, he may drink. If not, gently compress again.

7. Just continue to feed on the first side until the baby stops drinking.

8. If the baby stops drinking, take him off gently.

9. If the baby still wants some more milk, use the other breast and repeat the same process.

10. You may want to switch breasts a few times if you have sore nipples.

11. Look to always improve how you latch your baby.

Adopted Babies And Breast Feeding

Like your own baby, breast feeding an adopted baby is quite easy. You would produce a large enough amount of milk and it isn't complicated to do although it may be different to breast feeding a baby you are pregnant. There are generally two main objectives in this.

Firstly, is to get your baby to breast feed and the other is to simply produce enough breast milk. You need to be aware that there is more to breast feeding than simply giving the baby milk. Most mothers are happy to feed the baby nutritious milk, but the more important thing is the bond that the mothers would have with their baby that lasts an entire lifetime.

Many people feel that the introduction of bottles would interfere with breast feeding. This is true to a certain extent. Even the use of artificial nipples could interfere a great deal. If you can, make sure that the baby gets to your breasts as soon as possible after birth. The baby would require a good breast flow to stay attached and suck.

The moment you have adopted a baby, contact a lactation clinic to get your milk supply ready. You should keep in mind that you may not produce a full supply of milk for your baby. This is because you haven't gone through the whole pregnancy process.

However, don't feel discouraged by this. It is a normal thing. You have tried your very best to give your baby the best you can.

Breast Milk Jaundice

Jaundice is a situation where there is a buildup in the blood of the bilirubin. This comes about from the breakdown of the older red blood cells. It is very natural for red blood cells to break down although the formed bilirubin wouldn't normally cause jaundice as the liver would metabolize it and would get rid of it in the gut.

Due to the liver enzymes which metabolize the bilirubin becoming relatively immature, the newborn baby would become jaundiced during the first few days. From here, the newborn would have more red blood cells compared to adults and would break down at any time.

Breast milk jaundice is a condition where no one really knows the exact reason of it. To diagnose it, the baby would be at least a week old. The baby should be getting used to breast feeding alone while having a lot of bowel movement with passing of clean urine.

In such setting, the baby has breast milk jaundice. On certain occasion, urine infection or under-functioning of the baby's thyroid gland would peak at around 10-21 days and could last to up to 3 months.

Contrary to popular belief, breast milk jaundice is completely normal. Rarely do breastfeeding need to be stopped. If the baby is doing well on the breast milk, there isn't a good reason to stop or supplement with lactation aid.

Positioning For Breast Feeding

For certain mothers, breast feeding is a very natural process. However, there is a certain skill which is required for feeding successful and there is a correct technique to use. Positioning yourself wrongly is the biggest reason why feeding becomes unsuccessful.

In certain situations, this would even injure your nipples or breast. As you stroke the baby's cheek with your nipple, the baby would slowly open its mouth and head towards the nipple. From there, you should slowly push your nipples in so the baby could get a mouthful of your milk.

This position is called 'latching on'. Many women prefer to wear a nursing bra as it allows easier access to the breast compared to other bras. The length of feeding time would change; therefore, it is important for the mother to be very comfortable. Among the other position you can consider for your comfort includes:

- Upright position - This is a sitting position where your back is straight.
- Lying Down position - This is great when you are feeding the baby at night or for the mother who has a caesarean section.
- Mobile position - This is when the mother is carrying the baby in a sling/carrier. This easily allows the

mother to breastfeed while they are doing some work.

- On-Her-Back position - This position is when the mother is sitting slightly upright and is also a good position for tandem breast feeding

- On-Her-Side position - The mother and baby lie on their sides, on a bed.

- Hands And Knees position - The mother is on all fours while the baby is sucking underneath her. This is a very difficult position and is only done is certain circumstances when the baby find it difficult to suck.

Every position is different and you need to test each position in order to determine which the best position for you is.

Possible Complications From Breast Feeding

There are several possible complications from breast feeding. Among them include:

Sore Nipples

There are many mothers who complain about having tender nipples which make breast feeding a very painful and frustrating process. However, you need not worry because this condition is often just temporary. After some time, the nipples would toughen up and make breast feeding painless.

Many times, when the baby is positioned improperly or if they suck too hard, the breasts would be extremely sore. There are several ways of easing this discomfort. They include:

- Ensure that your baby is in the proper position. Having a properly positioned baby is the main cause of sore nipples.
- After the feeding, expose the breasts to air and protect them from clothing or other irritations.
- Once you have finished breast feeding, apply certain ultra-purified, medical-grade lanolin. Make sure to avoid petroleum jelly or other products with oil.

- After every breast feeding, if possible, wash your nipples with water and not soap.
- Teabags ran under cold water could provide some relief when it is placed on the nipples.
- Vary the breast feeding position every time you feed to make sure that different part of your nipple is compressed every time.

Clogged Milk Ducts

Small and red tender lumps on the tissue of your breasts are known as clogged milk ducts. Clogged milk ducts would cause the milk to back up and lead to an infection over a certain period.

The best method of unclogging these ducts is to make sure that you empty them as soon as you can. If you have a clogged breast, offer them first to your baby. Let your baby empty it as soon as possible. If there is still milk after that feeding, try to remove the remaining amount with your hand or a breast pump.

Besides that, try to keep the pressure off your breast ducts by ensuring that your bra isn't too tight. Clogged milk ducts could cause breast infection and it is normally due to several reasons.

This may be because empty breasts are completely out of milk, germs getting into your milk ducts through cracks in the nipples or decrease immunity in the mother due to inadequate nutrition or stress

Those mothers who have a breast infection have several symptoms. This includes severe pain, hardening breasts, redness of the breast, heat or even swelling. To treat breast infection you need to take a good bed rest, pain relievers, antibiotics, apply heat and drink more water. Even if you have a breast infection, don't stop your breast feeding.

When you empty your breast, you help to prevent the milk ducts from clogging. If, however, the pain is that bad that you couldn't feed, use a pump as you lie on a tub of warm water with your breasts floating comfortably in the water. If you do so, make sure that you don't use an electric pump.

You need to treat breast infection immediately or you risk the chance of swelling. This swelling is extremely painful and this includes swelling and throbbing. There would also be tenderness, heat and swelling. If your condition gets worse, the doctor may prescribe medication and even surgery in more severe cases.

Should You Breast Feed In Public

Any baby who is breast fed are very easy to comfort regardless of how busy your schedule is. However, most women feel worrisome about breast feeding in public. Nursing in public places would normally be worse that breast feeding itself. However, most people wouldn't even realize that you are breast feeding but other mothers who are doing the same thing.

Most women would try to find a way to breast feed unnoticeably. Some women would even ask a partner or a friend to stand in front of them while you lift your shirt. While breast feeding, your baby's body would cover most of your body and you could easily pull your shirt down to the face to ensure that the top of your breasts are covered.

While you are visiting someone, you may feel more comfortable leaving the room or finding a private area to breast feed. In many public places, restrooms are becoming even more baby-friendly and they now have separate changing table and chair. Some shopping malls offer special mother's room to ensure that the mom could easily breast feed their baby in private.

Another alternative method of doing this is to first pump your milk in the comfort of your home and then offering it from a bottle in public. This may be slightly difficult for your baby because they aren't used with artificial nipples from bottles. This would interfere with their breast feeding for a few weeks.

Breast feeding in public should depend a lot on testing what works best for you. It takes certain time for you to realize that this is a natural thing. With time, you would realize that it isn't that difficult to do. However, if you truly find it difficult to breast feed in certain locations, then you don't have to.

While feeding, you should make sure that you are comfortable as the baby would know that you are uncomfortable. The baby has an ability to know that you are uncomfortable and he would feel uncomfortable with breast feeding as well.

Toddlers And Breast Feeding

As more and more women choose to breast feed their babies, they are also finding that they enjoy it for an even longer period. They may enjoy it for more than just the few months that they have planned.

Some would even continue to breast feed their babies until they reach the toddler age, which is around the ages of 3 to 4 years old. This isn't unnatural as in many societies; toddlers are breast fed till they reach the ages of four years.

If the mother and baby enjoy breast feed, you shouldn't stop it. There is a myth that breast milk loses value after more than six months. This is totally untrue. Breast milk still contains fat, protein and many nutrients that all of us need, especially babies.

The most important thing is that breast milk would protect your baby against infection. It would also affect the maturing of the baby's immune systems and help other organs develop. It has been proven in the past few year from research that children who are still breast feeding have far less infections that children who aren't breast feeding.

Breast feeding your baby after six months of age is a very wise decision. Many people feel it isn't necessary, but if the mother and baby like it, then it shouldn't be a problem.

Without a doubt, breast milk is the best milk you could give to your baby.

Regardless of what other people tell you, breast feeding should only be stopped when the baby and mother stop enjoying it. Don't stop merely when someone else tells you to do it. Stop when you feel it's the right time.

Swollen Breasts

During the first few days after you have given birth, you would discover that your breasts are swollen, lumpy, tender and overly full. At times, this swelling would extend all the way to your armpit and you may have a slight fever.

The reason for this is because within 72 hours of birth, there would be an abundance of milk which would come in or become available to your baby. When this happens, the blood would flow to your breasts and the surrounding tissues would swell. This is the result of your swollen breasts.

However, not every mother would experience this swelling. While some women's breasts become slightly full, some would find their breast become very hard. Certain women would hardly notice the pain if they are busy with other things.

Don't worry about this condition too much. This is because this is a good sign that your body is producing milk to feed your baby. However, there are certain tips that could help you with this condition.

- Wear a supportive nursing bra, which isn't too tight.
- Avoid allowing your baby to suck when your areola is firm. This helps reduce the possibility of nipple

damage. Use a pump until your areola softens.

- Try to breast feed as often as you can, preferably 2-3 hours. Make sure that one breast is as soft as possible.

- Don't pump milk except when there is a need to soften your areola or when your baby has trouble latching on. If you pump excessively, this could lead to an over production of milk and prolonged swelling.

- Apply cold packs to your breasts for a short period to sooth the pain and relive swelling.

- Be positive. This is a very normal condition. It would pass after some time.

This condition passes very quickly. It would go away within 1-2 days. The best way is to nurse your baby. When you aren't breast feeding, it would only get worse.

Once the swelling has lessened, your breasts would become softer but still full of milk. During this period, you can and should continue to nurse. If not, the production of milk would drop and you should breast feed right from the very start. Keep an eye on your baby to spot when he is hungry and feed him appropriately.

Good Health And Proper Diet

It is important for the mother to maintain a healthy diet. This is because the baby relies a lot on the nutrition that he gets from the breast milk. What the mother eats would affect the nutrition that is in the breast milk.

If the baby is born large and grows fast, fat stored by the mother can be quickly depleted. Therefore, the mother would need to eat well to ensure that she is able to maintain a sufficient amount of milk.

This diet involves a very nutritious and high calorie diet after pregnancy. Even though a malnutrition mother can produce milk, the mother still needs to eat well in order to product milk which is rich with vitamins A, D, B6 and B12.

There are also added complications if the mother smokes. Having more than twenty cigarettes in a single day would reduce the milk supply. The infants would also have other symptoms like diarrhea, vomiting, rapid heart rate and restlessness throughout the day. There are also certain situations where the infants would have SIDS (Sudden Infant Death Syndrome), a condition when the babies are exposed to smoke.

Drinking a lot of alcohol could also affect the infant. If you breast feed, avoid alcohol at all cost. If the mother continues drinking and drinks excessively, the infant would be irritable, sleepless and grumpy. Although certain doctors would allow a few cups of alcohol a day, I would recommend not taking the risk. You should also look to avoid drinking excessive caffeine. Caffeine intake can be limited, but alcohol should be totally stopped.

After a healthy diet, this would ensure that your baby get the proper nutrients from breast feeding. This is a very important stage in the baby's growth. Don't take the risk.

Low Supply Of Milk

All mothers who breast feed would doubt if they have the adequate supply of milk. However, some mothers aren't able to produce the right amount of milk to meet the baby's needs.

According to many experts, insufficiency of milk is very rare. Many women think that they have insufficient milk supply but it isn't so. Mothers may feel such because the feel a lack of fullness in their breasts or if milk stop leaking from the nipples.

During growth spurts in the babies, they may want more milk than the norm. As such, the frequent feedings would leave your breasts less full. Because of it, the milk supply would lessen.

Another main factor which affects the production of milk is when the mother is ill or if she is consuming certain birth control pills. The best way for this condition is through doctor's care. Make sure that the baby gets frequent feedings and your nipple or milk ducts is healthy.

To ensure that this condition is alright, ask your doctor for advice. They would be able to run the tests needed to ensure everything in your body is fine. A low supply of breast milk would definitely affect your baby. Call your doctor immediately if your baby isn't gaining weight or losing weight quickly.

Better breast feeding techniques would help. In most cases, weight gain or loss indicates a very serious concern. In many cases, you can still breastfeed with a temporary decrease in milk supply.

Ask your doctor for the best ways to improve the milk supply. Among the main tips he would recommend is to actually eat healthy and have more frequent breast feeding. These two tips would go a long way to boosting your milk supply.

Nutrients In The Breast Milk

Until the age of four months of age, breast milk is the only food that your baby needs. With just breast milk alone for six months or better, the nutrient would be sufficient. In most circumstances, any other food or milk before 4-6 months isn't important. However, under certain circumstances, the baby needs to take more than just breast milk.

There are several valuable nutrients in the breast milk. Among the contents of the breast milk include:

- **Water** - Breast milk has more than 90% water. The baby therefore, wouldn't need to drink any extra water. Even if the baby isn't feeding well, extra water is still not needed. You should instead fix the breast feeding problems instead.

- **Iron** - Generally speaking, breast milk contain less iron than common formulas in the market. There are even formulas which are specially enriched with iron. Iron is valuable in that it gives the baby extra protection against certain infections. Iron which is found in breast milk can be utilized well by the baby, while it isn't available to bacteria. Don't delay the introduction of iron beyond the age of six months.

- **Vitamin D** - Breast milk don't contain a lot of Vitamin D. However, there is no need to worry because the baby would already store up Vitamin D while pregnancy. The baby would still be healthy without any supplements from Vitamin D. Unless you have a Vitamin D deficiency, you wouldn't need to take any supplements with Vitamin D. To get the right amount of Vitamin D, exposure to morning sun is more than sufficient.

Without a doubt, breast milk has all the nutrients which your baby needs in the first 6 months. After the first 6 months, only then should you introduce solid foods if he feels comfortable with it.

Baby Refuses To Breast Feed

At times, the baby may suddenly decide that he doesn't want to breast feed. The baby would move away from the breast and then toss his head from side to side. This is a very normal occurrence and could happen at any time. As such, there is probably no way of predicting when it happens. There are several reasons as to why this is happening.

Many times, this could be due to an infection, a thrust in the baby's mouth, teething or a sore head from vacuum delivery. Besides that, the use of dummies, teats or nipple shield may also contribute to this refusal.

Certain babies find it extremely difficult to feed from both a breast and a bottle as they are very different. Some babies become very confused. As such, try to avoid using any form of teats or dummies if you are looking to breast feed for the long term.

Some other times, the milk takes bitter. This could be because of antibiotics or if you use nipple creams. The baby would know if the milk tastes bitter. As such, don' force the baby to breast feed.

When you have such problems, always look to identify why the baby refuses to drink your breast milk. From then on, you can look to treat the cause of the problem. Be patient and gentle with your baby. Hold your baby next to you, so the baby could indicate to you as and when he wants to take the breast milk. He would know when it is enjoyable and comfortable.

The older babies may have shorter and fewer breast feeds while the younger would have longer and more frequent ones. This is different among all babies. Therefore, you shouldn't try to make the baby feed longer but allow the baby decide how long every individual feeding would be.

Breast Feeding And Work

Although you have continued work, you could still breastfeed. If you are someone who lives near to work or have an on-site daycare, you could easily continue breast feeding during your breaks. If you are someone who could work from home, this is even better. However, if you have to commute to work, you could still continue breast feeding.

If you still can't breast feed, there are two choices you could take. The first method is to keep your milk supply using an automatic electric breast pump. Save your breast milk and pass it to your baby sitter.

The second option is to simply use formulas. You can still breastfeed your baby, but the difference is that while you are working, the baby would be fed with formulas while fed with breast milk when you are around.

When you pump at work, this would stimulate your milk production. As such, you would have plenty of milk available when it is time to feed.

Collect the milk while you pump so your baby would have the nutritional benefits of breast milk even if you aren't there. Pumping is also an ideal method of making sure that you feel connected to your baby throughout the work day.

It may seem like a hassle, but many mothers find that the benefits far outweigh the inconvenience of breast feeding. There are several things you can do to ensure that breast feeding is as easy as possible. This includes having the right tools. They include:

- A fully electronic breast pump with a double collection kit so you can pump both your breast simultaneously.
- Access to a refrigerator or cooler to ensure that the milk is cool until you goes home.
- Breast pad to protect your clothes if your breast leaks.
- Bottles or bags for storing and collecting the milk.

Always ensure that you are used to pumping before you return to work. This is to make sure that you know what to expect and the feelings that come with it. From here, you would be confident with pumping at work when you know you can produce enough milk.

At work, you would want to have a place which is away from everyone else. This may be an empty office or room. This is to ensure that you are away from everyone else and you can have the quietness and tranquility so you can pump in peace. In most offices, you can easily find for such a spot.

You should try to pump every two to three hours if possible. Make sure that it doesn't affect your schedule at work. It would be better if you tell your superior about what you are doing. Most superiors would understand this. Once you have finished pumping, keep them in the bags or bottle. Then, clean yourself and go back to work. Once you are at home, you could feed the milk to your lovely baby.

Start Solid Foods For Your Baby

Until your baby reaches 4 months, your baby would only need breast milk. However, there would be a time where breast milk isn't sufficient to supply all your baby's nutrition needs. Around the age of six to nine months, the baby would start to require iron and this nutrition isn't sufficient from your breast milk.

Certain babies wouldn't start taking solid foods until they reach the ages of 9-12 months. However, many of them find it hard to take solid foods even at that age. When your child starts taking solid food, it is actually a development milestone as it means that your child is growing up. As a mother, you should definitely feel proud.

The best time to start taking solid food is when the baby starts showing interest. This is easy to notice as they would show interest in solid food which are placed on their parents' plate.

By the ages of around 5-6 months, the baby would actually try to grab the food from their parents' plate. When the baby starts reaching for food, it is usually the best indicator that you should start giving them some solid food.

At times, it would be better to start taking solid food earlier. When your baby is constantly hungry or he isn't gaining weight as he should, it is a good indicator that you should start feeding him solid food at an early age, even as early as three months.

Babies who are breast fed would generally digest solid foods better and earlier that babies which are fed with formulas. This is because breast milk contains certain enzymes which help digest proteins, starch and fats. Besides that, breast fed babies have different variety of tastes in the milk. These flavors would generally be passed on into the milk.

Once the baby starts taking solid foods around the ages of 5-6 months, there are certain things that you need to bear in mind. One of the main things is to avoid certain spicy foods or foods which are highly allergic. If your baby reaches for potato on your plate, you could let him have it if it isn't too hot.

Another method of deciding what food to give to him is to just give him the food he seems to be interested in. Let him enjoy the food and don't worry about it too much.

The quickest method of getting iron for your baby at the ages of 5-6 months is to give him meat. Infant cereals have iron and it is good for the baby, although it could be hard to be absorbed and cause the baby to be constipated.

Weaning From Breast Feeding

Weaning is when you baby has stopped depending on breast milk. When your baby has stopped breast milk and gets all of his nutrients from other sources, he is considered weaned. Some babies are weaned from the milk bottle as well. However, this term is more often referred when the baby has stopped breast feeding.

When it is the mother who decides to stop breast feeding, it would require lots of patience and can take a bit of time. This depends on the age of your toddler and how well your child adjusts. This isn't the same experience for everybody.

Weaning is something difficult. It is a long goodbye, filled with a lot of emotions and could be incredibly painful. However, this doesn't signal the end of intimacy between the mother and child. What this simply means is that you are just replaced breast feeding with other forms of nutrition.

It is hard to decide when to start weaning. The mother is the best judge for this. There isn't a deadline unless the mother and child are ready to wean. The normal recommended time for this is normally one year. There isn't a right and wrong as to the best time for weaning.

Regardless of what age your child is, you should proceed slowly. Experts say that you should never abruptly withhold your breast from your child. This can cause a lot of trauma for your baby. There are certain methods that you could try during this process. It includes:

- **Try To Skip A Feeding** - Just skip a feeding and see the reaction from your baby. Instead, offer your baby a bottle of milk. You could simply substitute by using a bottle of your pumped breast milk, formula or even cow's milk. As you slowly reduce the feedings, your child would be better able to adjust to these changes.

- **Follow The Feeding With A Healthy Snack** - This depends on the age. Try it and sees if your baby likes it.

- **Shorten The Feeding Time** - You could also start by shortening the time your child is on the breast. If you normally feed him for ten minutes, cut short and feed him for only five minutes.

- **Postpone The Feeding** - You could postpone those feedings if you are feeding the baby a few times a day. This is a great method if you have an older child who understands what you are saying. Tell him that you will feed him later and then distract him. He may totally forget about it.

If you tried hard and weaning just doesn't seem to happen, perhaps the time isn't right. Just wait slightly longer to see what happens. Weaning is pretty much a decision you make with your child. You need to decide on this based on the reaction of your baby.

Resource 1 - How To Wean

Weaning is a problem that many mothers have. When it comes to weaning, there are several issues that the mother has to consider.

Weaning from breastfeeding is not simply done by abruptly quitting breastfeeding. There's more to consider, including:

- **Make sure my baby doesn't feel abandoned by their mom during weaning.**
- Help baby adjust to the new way of taking milk (either formula or expressed breast milk).
- **How to stop lactation, avoiding complications like pain, engorgement, and infection.**
- What to do when baby is having a hard time switching.
- **How to wean baby from night feedings - and help baby sleep through the night.**

For more information on this, go to:
http://weaning.wellbeingvalley.com/

Resource 2 - Breast Feeding Food

What if there was a food that was <u>perfectly suited to your baby's delicate digestive system</u>; that could offer both **immediate and long term protection** against bacteria, viruses and serious illness such as cancer; that didn't harm the environment to *produce and was readily available at virtually no financial cost to you?!*

For more information about this amazing food, go to:

http://breastfeeding.wellbeingvalley.com/